BLADDER CANCER

The Ultimate Patient Survival Manual

By

Angel B. Maurice

Copyright © by Angel B. Maurice 2023.All rights reserved.

Before this document is duplicated or reproduced in any manner, the publisher's consent must be gained. Therefore, the contents within can neither be stored electronically, transferred, nor kept in a database. Neither in Part nor full can the document be copied, scanned, faxed, or retained without approval from the publisher or creator.

Table of Contents

Introduction

Millions of people all over the world face a strong foe which is bladder cancer. The bladder is a hollow organ that stores urine until it is expelled from the body. Its lining can get infected with this complex disease. While bladder cancer may not get as much press as other malignancies, it nevertheless has a significant impact and presents considerable hurdles.

The purpose of this book is to serve as a comprehensive resource for learning about and dealing with bladder cancer. This resource is meant to equip anyone with knowledge about bladder cancer, whether you are a new patient, a caregiver, a worried loved one, or just curious about the disease.

First, we'll examine some of the most fundamental information on bladder cancer. We'll talk about the many forms of bladder cancer, what they look like, and what causes or contributes to them. By the time you finish this chapter, you will have a firm grasp of the nature of the illness.

The key to effective treatment is oftentimes early discovery. From taking a patient's medical history and conducting a physical exam to doing additional tests and treatments, this chapter will show you all you need to know about the diagnostic process. In addition, you'll gain knowledge about cancer staging, an important procedure for assessing the discasc's scvcrity before beginning treatment.

Bladder cancer treatments are not one-size-fits-all. Cancer patients have a wide range of treatment options depending on several factors, including cancer type, stage, and the patient's general condition. Surgery, chemotherapy, radiation therapy, immunotherapy, and targeted therapy are only some of the options discussed in this chapter. The importance of clinical trials in advancing our treatment options for bladder cancer, and how these developments have been implemented, will be discussed.

Although receiving therapy can improve one's chances of survival, it is not without its share of difficulties. Many patients having treatment for bladder cancer report unpleasant side effects, such as decreased energy and nausea or altered bladder control. Methods for minimizing the impact of these unwanted effects on your daily life during and after treatment are covered in this section.

A person's mental health, relationships, and ability to go about their everyday activities can all be negatively impacted by bladder cancer. In this chapter, we'll talk about how to deal with bladder cancer holistically, from the food you eat to the activities you participate in the people who support you emotionally to the changes in your daily routine that can make a big difference.

Treatment is only the beginning of the process. In fact, for many people, this marks the start of a new stage: survivorship. What to expect following treatment, why it's crucial to have regular checkups, and how to move forward with optimism and strength will all be covered.

Treatment is never as good as prevention. In this chapter, we will discuss lifestyle modifications that can improve bladder health and decrease your risk of developing bladder cancer.

You don't have to deal with bladder cancer alone, and knowledge is a potent weapon. To aid you on your journey, we will present a plethora of resources, such as support groups, organizations, websites, books, and a glossary of terms.

Although there are many obstacles to overcome when fighting bladder cancer, it is possible to do so with the right information, attitude, and community. your book is here to help you face your sickness head-on by providing you with direction, resources, and encouragement. Our future is bright if we work together to learn more about bladder cancer, develop better treatments, and eliminate the disease altogether.

Chapter 1

Cancer of the Bladder: An Overview

Having bladder cancer is a frightening reality for millions of individuals throughout the world. Understanding what bladder cancer is, how it progresses, and why early identification and care are critical is essential for a successful journey.

Bladder cancer: what is it?

Bladder cancer develops from cells in the bladder, the organ that collects and stores pee until it is eliminated. The urinary system, which includes the bladder, which looks like a tiny hollow balloon, is responsible for flushing waste out of the body. Bladder cancer develops when malignant cells start to multiply inside the bladder's lining.

Bladder Cancer Subtypes

There is no universally effective treatment for bladder cancer. Many different kinds exist, and each has its unique set of traits. Urothelial carcinoma, sometimes called transitional cell carcinoma, is the most frequent form of bladder cancer. The vast majority of bladder cancers start in the cells that line the inside of the bladder.

Squamous cell carcinoma and adenocarcinoma are two other kinds of bladder cancer that are much less prevalent. Chronic irritation or inflammation of the bladder, as seen with urinary tract infections or long-term catheter use, is a common cause of squamous cell carcinoma. However, adenocarcinoma is rare because the disease develops in the glandular cells of the bladder.

Factors and Root Causes of Risk

Knowing the various causes and risk factors for bladder cancer is important for early detection and prevention. Although the precise origin of bladder cancer is unknown, some risk factors have been identified:

1. Cigarette smoking is the single most important risk factor for developing bladder cancer. Tobacco smoke contains several compounds that can be taken into the bloodstream and concentrated in the urine, where they can cause damage to the bladder.
2. The majority of instances of bladder cancer occur in adults over the age of 55, and as a result, the risk rises with age.
3. When comparing the sexes, males have a higher risk of developing bladder cancer.

4. Chemicals used in the textile, rubber, leather, and dye industries, among others, may raise the risk of bladder cancer if workers are exposed to them on the job.

5. Conditions that irritate or inflame the bladder over time, such as repeated UTIs or the use of indwelling catheters, may increase vulnerability.

6. Radiation therapy and some types of chemotherapy may modestly raise the chance of developing bladder cancer in patients who have undergone those treatments in the past.

7. A higher risk may be present if there is a personal or family history of bladder cancer.

Those who are aware of the probable causes and risk factors can take measures to lessen their vulnerability, such as giving up harmful habits like smoking and adopting a healthier lifestyle.

Indicators and Signs

Understanding the signs and symptoms of bladder cancer is essential for early detection and treatment. Common symptoms include:

• Hematuria (blood in the urine).
Rapid urination
• Urinary discomfort
Pain in the lower back
• Abdominal pain
Lack of motivation to eat

If you encounter any of these symptoms, it is essential to see a doctor for a thorough evaluation because they may also be signs of other disorders affecting the urinary tract.

Bladder cancer is discussed in further depth in this book, along with its diagnosis, treatment choices, coping methods, and support networks. If people are aware of the symptoms of bladder cancer and how to treat them, they will be better equipped to deal with the disease and improve their quality of life.

Chapter2

Bladder Cancer: Diagnosis and Staging

Bladder cancer is diagnosed after a thorough patient history and physical examination as well as a battery of diagnostic testing. The presence, type, and stage of bladder cancer must be determined at this point for proper treatment planning and prognosis.

Examination and Medical History

In many cases, a diagnosis of bladder cancer begins with a thorough medical history and physical examination. You should expect to be asked about your symptoms, risk factors, and family history of cancer during your first appointment with your doctor. To check for abnormalities in the surrounding organs, they will also perform a physical examination, which may involve a pelvic exam in women and a rectal exam in men.

Tests for Detecting Bladder Cancer

Several different diagnostic tests and procedures can be used to either confirm or rule out the presence of bladder cancer:

1. The initial stage in the cytology of the urinary tract is usually the microscopic examination of a urine sample for the presence of cancer cells or other abnormalities. Although useful, urine cytology may not always reveal bladder cancer in its earliest stages.
2. One of the most important tests for detecting bladder cancer is a procedure called a cystoscopy. This test involves inserting a thin, flexible tube (cystoscope) equipped with a camera into the bladder via the urethra. This

paves the way for the doctor to inspect the inside of the bladder and spot any tumors or other abnormalities.

3. Studies of the patient's internal organs and lymph nodes, as well as any distant organs, may be scanned with a CT scanner, MRI scanner, or ultrasound machine to evaluate the full scope of the cancer and whether or not it has progressed beyond the bladder.

4. When cystoscopy or imaging reveals a questionable spot, a biopsy is often conducted to confirm or rule out the diagnosis. During a biopsy, a small piece of bladder tissue is removed for microscopic analysis. This biopsy is useful for establishing a diagnosis of cancer and determining its subtype.

Cancer of the Bladder Progression

After a diagnosis of bladder cancer has been made, determining the disease's stage is essential. Cancer staging involves determining the disease's extent and whether or not it has spread to other organs. The prognosis and subsequent course of treatment are heavily dependent on accurate staging.

Tumor, Lymph Nodes, and Metastasis (TNM) is the standard approach for staging bladder cancer.

The original bladder tumor's size and spread are assessed at Stage T (Tumor). The range is from Ta (limited to the lining of the bladder) to T4b (extensive invasion into neighboring structures).
N (Lymph Nodes): Determines if cancer has spread to lymph nodes in the area. Without lymph node involvement (N0), lymph node involvement (N1, N2, or N3) increases.

In this stage, we look for evidence that the cancer has spread to other organs (metastasized). Disease has not spread to other parts of the body (M0), but has spread elsewhere (M1). Depending on how far the cancer has spread and how well the inner lining has been able to protect it, the cancer may be classified as early (stage 0) or late (stage IV) for staging purposes. Tumors diagnosed at an early stage of bladder cancer are typically surgically removed, whereas those at a later stage may require a mix of treatments including chemotherapy, radiation therapy, and immunotherapy.

Overall, a thorough medical history, physical exam, diagnostic testing, and staging assessments are required to correctly diagnose and stage bladder cancer. To improve the likelihood of successful treatment and long-term survival, an early and precise diagnosis is crucial.

Chapter 3

Bladder cancer treatment options

Factors such as the type of disease, the stage of the illness, the patient's overall health, and the patient's preferences all play a role in the therapy of bladder cancer. To properly tackle the condition, a complete treatment strategy may generally incorporate multiple methods. In this article, we'll take a look at all the different ways bladder cancer can be treated.

1. Surgery

Depending on the stage and degree of the disease, a variety of surgical procedures may be used to treat bladder cancer.

• Transurethral resection of bladder tumor (TURBT): a cystoscope put via the urethra is commonly used to remove non-invasive tumors in early-stage bladder cancer. The diagnostic and staging potential of this minimally invasive technique is also being explored.

When bladder cancer is localized to one location, a surgeon can remove that area of the bladder while leaving the rest of the bladder intact and functioning.

In more severe cases, a surgeon may opt to remove the bladder in its entirety, a procedure known as a radical cystectomy. In some cases, a urinary diversion (ileal conduit or neobladder) may be necessary for this treatment.

2. Chemotherapy

Chemotherapy can be injected intravenously (IV) or inserted directly into the bladder (intravesical chemotherapy). Chemotherapy can be used as a main treatment for advanced or metastatic bladder cancer, in addition to or instead of surgery.

3. Therapy Radiation

Radiation therapy involves exposing cancer cells to X-rays or other forms of high-energy radiation to kill them. It can be used either on its own or in tandem with other therapies. Internal radiation (brachytherapy) involves inserting radioactive materials into the bladder rather than using an external beam to treat the bladder.

4. Immunotherapy

Intravesical immunotherapy, in which drugs like Bacillus Calmctte-Guérin (BCG) are injected into the bladder to treat non-invasive bladder cancer, is widely utilized. Checkpoint inhibitors (e.g., pembrolizumab, mepolizumab) have shown potential in blocking proteins that hinder immune cells from attacking cancer cells and hence in treating advanced bladder cancer.

5. Aimed Treatment

Drugs used in targeted therapy are developed to attack cancer's underlying molecular abnormalities. In circumstances where standard chemotherapy has failed to control the disease, targeted treatments have been approved for the treatment of advanced bladder cancer.

6. New Treatments and Human Studies

Treatment options for bladder cancer are constantly improving because of ongoing research and clinical trials. Clinical trials are a way to gain access to new medicines, some of which may be more beneficial or have fewer negative effects than standard care.

The medical staff at your facility can assist you in identifying potential clinical trial choices.

7. Care That Encourages

Patient comfort and quality of life are prioritized during bladder cancer therapy with the help of supportive care. The emotional toll of illness and treatment can be mitigated with the help of professionals in the fields of pain management, nutrition, and psychology.

8. Hospice and Palliative Medicine

Patients with advanced bladder cancer are a prime target for palliative treatment because of the severity of their condition. The primary goals of this treatment are symptom management, pain reduction, and improvement of the patient's overall quality of life.

The stage and grade of your bladder cancer, as well as your general health and personal preferences, will all play a role in determining the best course of therapy. Urologists, oncologists, radiation therapists, and nurses are just some of the members of the healthcare team who work closely with patients to build individualized treatment programs.

In conclusion, the treatment of bladder cancer is an evolving subject with a wide variety of approaches that can be adapted to meet the needs of individual patients. To effectively attack bladder cancer and improve long-term outcomes, patients should engage closely with healthcare providers to make educated decisions about the optimal treatment strategy.

Chapter 4

Treatment for Bladder Cancer: Coping with Adverse Effects

Although helpful in curing the disease, bladder cancer treatment frequently causes several unpleasant side effects that can compromise a patient's quality of life. To achieve the greatest potential outcome and general well-being during and after treatment, it is crucial to comprehend and proactively manage these adverse effects.

Negative Effects of Treating Bladder Cancer

1. Alterations in urine Function
   Alterations in urine function are among the most often reported adverse effects of treatment for bladder cancer. Adjusting to new urination habits or the

need for a urinary diversion after surgery is common. Patients undergoing intravesical or radiation therapy may have urine urgency, frequency, and discomfort.

2. Weakness: Tiredness is a common reaction to cancer therapy. Chemotherapy and radiation therapy are two situations in which this can become very noticeable. Keeping a healthy diet, drinking enough of water, and doing some mild exercise when you can are all great ways to fight weariness.

3. Nausea and vomiting are common side effects of chemotherapy medications. Medications to treat these symptoms can be prescribed by your healthcare provider. Eating frequent and light meals may also be beneficial.

4. Discomfort and pain are possible side effects of surgery or radiation

treatment. Strategies for managing pain, such as medication or localized therapy, can be suggested by your medical team. Discussing your pain levels honestly with your healthcare providers allows them to better tailor their care to your needs.

5. Radiation therapy to the pelvis has been linked to changes in bowel habits, such as diarrhea and constipation. Eating a high-fiber diet and drinking lots of water both can help with symptom management. It is important to talk to your healthcare team before utilizing any OTC medications, even if they promise to relieve your symptoms.

6. Irritation or sensitivity of the skin in the treated area is a potential side effect of external beam radiation therapy. You can reduce skin-related adverse effects by using mild skincare products and following your doctor's advice.

7. The psychological and emotional effects of a cancer diagnosis and therapy cannot be understated. It's not unusual to experience emotions like worry, sadness, and terror. Counseling, therapy, or joining a support group can be quite helpful at times like these.

Methods of Coping and Consoling

Medical treatment and self-care are both necessary for symptom management during bladder cancer treatment.

1. Honesty and openness in communicating with your healthcare staff is essential. They need to know about your side effects so that they can make adjustments to your treatment and give you the care you need.
2. Maintenance of energy, nausea, and regular bowel movements are all aided

by a healthy diet. If you need specific advice on what to eat, see a nutritionist.

3. Maintaining an adequate fluid intake is essential, especially if you're experiencing dizziness, nausea, or vomiting. Your healthcare practitioner should be consulted regarding your fluid consumption as there may be restrictions associated with your therapy.

4. Don't be ashamed to ask for help if you're in agony. Your healthcare staff may suggest drugs or other methods for dealing with your pain.

5. Exercising: Light, low-impact activities like walking or yoga are great ways to fight weariness and feel better in general. Before beginning any new workout program, it is important to have your doctor's approval.

6. It is critical to address the psychological effects of bladder cancer

treatment. Participate in therapy, counseling, or a support group. It often helps to talk about how you're feeling with people you care about.

7. Radiation therapy can cause skin irritation, so it's important to use the products and methods recommended by your doctor if you're experiencing any discomfort.

8. Palliative care is a type of medical care that focuses on easing the suffering of patients with terminal illnesses, such as advanced bladder cancer.

Keep in mind that reactions to medications might vary from patient to patient, and that what helps some may hurt others. It's crucial to collaborate closely with your healthcare team to create a specialized plan for dealing with side effects that take into account your specific requirements and situation.

Coping with treatment-related side effects is an important part of the cancer care process. Patients can better manage therapy and keep up their quality of life while fighting bladder cancer if they anticipate and seek help with these obstacles.

Chapter 5

Survival While Having Bladder Cancer

A diagnosis of bladder cancer can alter one's life in profound ways, yet it need not determine one's identity or future prospects. You can keep living a full life while having this illness if you have access to the resources, knowledge, and attitude you need.

Nutritional Diet

During and after treatment for bladder cancer, eating a healthy, well-rounded diet is crucial to your health and well-being. Because of the potential for treatment-related side effects on appetite and digestion, here are some dietary considerations to keep in mind:

1. Staying hydrated is especially important after surgery or when experiencing a change in urinary habits, so make sure to drink lots of fluids. Talk to your healthcare providers about your individual fluid consumption requirements.
2. Whole grains, fruits, and vegetables are all great examples of fiber-rich foods that can help you control gastrointestinal movements. A diet high in fiber can help with both diarrhea and constipation.
3. Lean Protein: Consume lean protein sources including chicken, fish, beans, and tofu to aid in muscle repair and maintenance.
4. Caffeine, alcohol, and spicy meals are just a few examples of bladder irritants that should be avoided. Consider regulating or avoiding irritants and

paying attention to how your body reacts to various foods.

5. Consider meeting with a qualified dietician for tailored nutritional advice that takes into consideration your individual needs and any constraints imposed by your course of treatment.

Health and Fitness

Keeping active and taking care of one's health is essential for dealing with bladder cancer and its symptoms.

1. Low-Impact Exercise: Activities like walking, yoga, and swimming are great examples of mild, low-impact workouts that can help you feel better in many ways. Before beginning any new workout program, it is important to have your doctor's approval.

2. Anxiety Management Getting a cancer diagnosis can be traumatic. Mindfulness, meditation, and the use of support groups are all strategies for dealing with stress and keeping a healthy perspective.
3. Get plenty of good sleep to help your body repair and rejuvenate. Create a relaxing space to sleep in and stick to a regular bedtime routine.

Psychological and Emotional Encouragement

Bladder cancer can have a devastating psychological effect. It's crucial to look for help:

1. Therapy & Counseling: If you anticipate experiencing anxiety, despair, or any other emotional issues

on your trip, you may wish to explore these options.

2. Joining a support group for people with bladder cancer is a great way to meet people who understand what you're going through and receive encouragement and advice.

3. Keep the lines of communication open and honest with those you care about. If you tell your loved ones about how you're feeling, they can help ease your worries.

Mode of Living Shifts

Adjustments to your routine may be necessary when dealing with bladder cancer:

1. If you've had surgery or treatment that altered your urine function, you may have to learn to do things differently.

Take your time while you figure out how to adapt to these alterations.

2. Maintaining excellent bladder hygiene is important for preventing urinary tract infections (UTIs) and other bladder-related problems. Always drink plenty of water and use the restroom frequently.

3. Attend all scheduled follow-up appointments with your healthcare provider so that they can track your progress and handle any issues as soon as possible.

Connections and Helping Hands

Managing bladder cancer is not something you have to do alone. Count on your community for help:

1. Talk to your loved ones about what you want and what worries you. They

intend to be there for you and offer assistance as you go through this.

2. If you are fortunate enough to have a caregiver, it is imperative that you provide them with the necessary resources and assistance. They may benefit from attending a support group or talking to a therapist because providing care can be emotionally taxing.

Strength and optimism

Despite the difficulties, many people who have been diagnosed with bladder cancer go on to live happy and productive lives. Keep in mind that there are better options and outcomes for treatment now than ever before. If you want a better and healthier future, you must keep your hope and resilience strong.

Overall, a holistic approach that prioritizes one's physical and mental health as well as the love and support of friends and family is necessary for a life with bladder cancer. You may keep your optimism and resolve in the face of bladder cancer by being proactive about your diet, maintaining a healthy lifestyle, getting emotional support, and staying connected with your healthcare team.

Chapter 6

Survival Rates and Long-Term Monitoring Following Bladder Cancer Therapy

Even though beating bladder cancer is a major victory, your life's journey is far from over. To ensure your sustained health and to watch for any possible recurrence or complications after treatment, it is crucial to pay attention to survivorship and follow-up care.

Aftercare in Daily Life

Adjustment and introspection are common after therapy for bladder cancer. Feelings of relaxation, appreciation, doubt, and even dread are all possible reactions. Here are some important things to think about as you begin your post-treatment life: Your healthcare team will plan follow-up appointments at regular intervals to check in on your progress and evaluate your health as a whole. At these visits, you can ask questions, voice concerns, and get any necessary imaging or testing done. Emotional complexity post-treatment makes coping with them a priority. Having anxiety, despair, or a fear of a recurrence is common among cancer survivors. Therapy, counseling, or participation in a support group can help you deal with these feelings. Third, modify your lifestyle to improve your health by eating better, getting more exercise, and ditching bad habits like smoking. Your health and well-being as a whole may benefit from these adjustments. Maintaining proper bladder hygiene reduces the likelihood of urinary tract infections (UTIs) and other bladder-related problems. Keep drinking water, using the restroom frequently, and doing whatever else your doctor tells you to do.

Monitoring and Checkups regularly

Care after treatment for bladder cancer has ended is vital. Your healthcare team will create a unique plan for your follow-up treatment based on your individual needs. Included in this strategy are:1. Physical tests: Routine physical tests, particularly pelvic exams, to track any symptoms or changes.Cystoscopy 2: Routine cystoscopy examinations to view the bladder's interior and look for recurrence. These checkups may be scheduled at varying intervals depending on your specific needs. Third, periodic imaging examinations, including as CT scans, MRIs, or ultrasounds, may be performed to assess the urinary tract and nearby organs, depending on your stage and risk factors.4.Urine tests: Routine urine tests to detect anomalies, such as cancer cells, are performed.5.Blood Tests: Blood tests to evaluate general health and identify kidney or other organ dysfunction.6. Biopsies: Sometimes your doctor will want to confirm or rule out the presence of malignant cells by taking a sample of tissue.

Wellness and Method of Living

Survivors of bladder cancer need to focus on more than just medical monitoring to become better:1.Nutrition: Maintain a diet that emphasizes a variety of colorful produce, lean meats, and whole grains. If you have nutritional questions or concerns, you should talk to a nutritionist. Maintaining muscle strength, increasing vitality, and fostering general well-being all require frequent physical activity. Before beginning any new workout program, it is important to have your doctor's approval. To keep your mind and heart in good shape, try some stress-busting activities like yoga, meditation, or mindful eating 4. If you smoke, stopping is one of the best things you can do for your long-term health and to lessen the likelihood that cancer will return.

Recurrence Anxiety

A common worry for many who have overcome bladder cancer is that it will return. It's human to worry, but finding a happy medium between worrying and living is key. Talk to your healthcare providers about your fears, and see if there are any resources they may recommend to help you cope, such as mindfulness exercises or counseling.

Resilience, hope, and constant attention to one's own needs are the hallmarks of the road to survival after treatment for bladder cancer. You can confidently and optimistically face the world as a bladder cancer survivor by actively engaging in regular follow-up care, keeping a healthy lifestyle, and addressing emotional and psychological needs. Your healthcare staff and support system are there to help you every step of the way, so don't feel alone.

Chapter 7

Reducing Bladder Cancer Risks and Preventing It

Although several factors can increase your risk of developing bladder cancer, there are also things you can do to improve your bladder's health and lower that risk. You can lessen your chances of getting this condition by taking preventative measures.

1.Tobacco smoke contains chemicals that are absorbed into the bloodstream and then expelled in the urine, putting the bladder in danger of being exposed to these chemicals.

The primary method of lowering one's risk of bladder cancer is giving up smoking. Get help from a smoking cessation program or a medical expert if you're having trouble kicking the habit.

2. Stay away from potentially dangerous chemicals

Chemicals used in the textile, leather, rubber, and dyeing industries have been associated with an elevated risk of bladder cancer among workers in these fields. Following safety practices, using protective equipment, and abiding by workplace safety guidelines can reduce your exposure to harmful chemicals at work.

3. Keep Drinking Water

Keeping yourself adequately hydrated can lower your risk of bladder cancer by reducing the concentration of possible carcinogens in your urine. Maintain a healthy hydration intake throughout the day. Adequate water intake is linked to better general health.

4. Nutrition and Diet

Vitamins, minerals, and antioxidants included in a diet rich in fruits and vegetables help maintain general health and may lower the chance of developing bladder cancer. Antioxidant-rich meals, such as those rich in vitamin C and beta-carotene, have been suggested to have protective effects by certain research. You can get these essential nutrients by eating a wide variety of fruits and vegetables of different colors.

Reduce your alcohol intake.

The chance of developing bladder cancer is thought to rise in tandem with alcohol intake levels. Moderate alcohol intake, consistent with safe drinking recommendations, is encouraged.

Take Care of Your Weight6.

An increased risk of developing bladder cancer has been associated with obesity and being overweight. Aim for a healthy weight by eating well and staying active regularly. Maintaining a healthy weight is crucial not just for avoiding bladder cancer but for living a long and happy life.

Constant bladder infections: 7. Treatment

A higher chance of developing bladder cancer, and in particular squamous cell carcinoma, has been linked to a history of chronic or recurring urinary tract infections (UTIs). Good hygiene, adequate fluid intake, and frequent urination are all recommended to reduce the risk of UTIs. Talk to your doctor about treatment options and ways to avoid future infections if you suffer from recurrent UTIs.

8. Scheduled Health Exams

The detection of bladder cancer at an early, more curable stage can be aided by routine medical examinations. Talk to your doctor if you're worried about potential health consequences from variables like smoking or chemical exposure in your past. They can provide you with specific recommendations for tests and precautions to take.

Although some risk factors for bladder cancer, such as age, gender, and family history, are out of your hands, you can take steps to greatly lower that risk. You can significantly reduce your risk of developing bladder cancer by making healthy lifestyle choices including giving up smoking, reducing your exposure to toxic chemicals, drinking plenty of water, eating a balanced diet, and getting regular exercise. Early detection and rapid intervention, if necessary, depend on regular checkups and open discussions with your healthcare provider. Always keep in mind that the best way to ensure your bladder's and general health is through preventative measures.

Conclusion

Knowledge, early identification, and aggressive management can help people with bladder cancer face this difficult and complex disease with strength and optimism. The many sides of bladder cancer have been covered in this book, from the disease's origins and diagnosis to possible treatments, side effects, survivorship, and preventative strategies.

The first step in treating a condition is having a firm grasp on what causes it. Although everybody is at risk for developing bladder cancer, those who smoke, those who work in certain environments, and those who have a family history of the disease are at a higher risk. Timely treatment requires prompt diagnosis, which can be achieved through diagnostic procedures such as urine testing, cystoscopy, and imaging studies.

Surgery, chemotherapy, radiation treatment, immunotherapy, and targeted therapy are only some of the possibilities for treating bladder cancer. Cancer kind, cancer stage, and the patient's general condition all play a role in determining the best course of treatment. The quality of life during and after treatment can be enhanced by taking steps to manage treatment-related side effects and adopting a healthy lifestyle.

Survival is a distinct stage in the fight against bladder cancer. Maintaining mental and psychological health and adjusting to the possibility of a change in urine function are all part of this aftercare process. To fully embrace life after bladder cancer, it is important to seek help from medical professionals, therapists, support groups, and loved ones.

Individuals can reduce their risk of acquiring bladder cancer through the use of prevention and risk-reduction techniques. Proactive measures can dramatically minimize the incidence of this disease, including giving up smoking, limiting exposure to dangerous chemicals, staying hydrated, having a balanced diet, and treating persistent bladder infections.

Although there are many obstacles to overcome when dealing with bladder cancer, the disease is still treatable with the right attitude, a strong support system, and a thorough awareness of the disease. This book is a helpful friend in your battle against bladder cancer, providing information, direction, and encouragement. Our collective efforts will perhaps one day lead to a world where bladder cancer is fully understood, successfully treated, and eventually defeated.

www.ingramcontent.com/pod-product-compliance
Lightning Source LLC
Chambersburg PA
CBHW070727260726
48660CB00007B/2757